Bell's Palsy Natural Treatments
and Cures

ISBN: 1-4528-6934-0
ISBN-13: 9781452869346

Bell's Palsy Natural Treatments and Cures

Johnathan Porter

2010

Disclaimer

This information within this book contains information on supplements, studies and treatment protocol suggestions. Do NOT construe this as medical advice. Medical advice can only be given by a licensed professional who has had a chance to personally observe you and understands your condition, position and objectives.

The information presented here is not intended to replace the attention or advice of a physician or other health care professional. It talks about health issues in general for a 'statistical' user, not you as a specific user, and is not referring to your specific healthcare issue. Anyone who wishes to embark on any dietary, drug, exercise, supplement or other lifestyle change intended to prevent or treat a specific disease or condition should first consult with and seek clearance from a qualified healthcare practitioner.

This information has not been reviewed or approved by the FDA. It is provided under First Amendment rights for educational and communication purposes only, and should not be construed as personal medical advice. The FDA has ruled that only a healthcare professional can diagnose a medical problem—and, from their perspective, that may include you, the person who actually has the problem. Therefore, this information and any products presented along with it, should be used only to inform yourself about available choices in conjunction with consultation of a healthcare professional.

Table of Contents

Chapter 1
What Is Bell's Palsy?

Bell's Palsy is a condition that causes the facial muscles to weaken so that one or both sides of an individual's face become paralyzed. You can be fine one day, go to sleep at night and wake up the next day with Bell's Palsy facial paralysis, and have had no prior warning whatsoever.

The typical symptoms of Bell's Palsy include muscle weakness/paralysis, having an asymmetrical smile, droopy appearance, the inability to close your eye(s) completely, excessive tearing and or dry eye(s), facial pain, facial swelling, loss of the wrinkling on the forehead, facial spasms/contractures, drooling from the mouth, nose runs, food caught in cheek, hyperacussis (sensitivity to sounds) or pain in/near the ear, difficulties of speech, loss of taste, and occasional difficulty in swallowing.

Typically,

- About 50% of patients experience pain in the mastoid region of the face
- Two-thirds have problems with their tear flow
- 80% show a reduced sense of taste
- Dry eyes are a prevalent condition

There are many physical symptoms associated with Bell's Palsy, but they usually vary amongst individuals in accordance with the degree and location of the nerve damage involved with the condition.

The facial paralysis of Bell's Palsy usually occurs on just one side of the face (a situation called "unilateral palsy") but it can occur on both sides. It occurs usually without warning and can happen to anyone, at any time. It is unusual to see Bell's Palsy in children less than 10 years old and the average age of sufferers seems to be around 37 years. Older people succumb to it with a slightly higher frequency than younger people. About 40,000 Americans get it per year.

Bell's Palsy[1] is caused by trauma to the 7th cranial nerve in the head (though other nerves can be temporarily irritated). The best science today suggests that the trauma is caused by the herpes simplex virus, though the actual cause of the condition is unknown. While there are many possible causes for the condition, the DNA for the HSV-1 virus has been detected in 86% of facial nerve ganglia of persons who have had Bell's Palsy, compared to only 43% of controls (Linder et al, 2005).

Nevertheless, there are a wide variety of other possible causes behind Bell's Palsy including diabetes, Lyme disease, sarcoidosis, HIV infection, and various cancers or tumors. When a doctor is trying to make a diagnosis, he first tries to rule out these possibilities as well as high blood pressure, acute otitis media, chronic ear disease, and chronic systemic, neurological and metabolic disorders. The real distinguishing characteristic of Bell's Palsy is that unlike these other conditions it comes on suddenly. There is no specific test for Bell's Palsy.

Statistics suggest that Bell's Palsy happens to approximately .025% of the population...which is 25 of every 100,000 people every year. The incidence of Bell's Palsy in males and females, as well as racially, is approximately equal. Bilateral Bell's Palsy is rare but possible, and accounts for less than 1% of all cases. The incidents occurring on either side of the face are approximately the same in number. The percentage of left or right side cases also remains equal for any recurrences.

The most recent studies suggest the recurrence rate is between 5-9% with an average recurrence time span of 10 years. Recurrence tends to cluster in families as well as in diabetics. To me this suggests a biochemical workup on sufferers (a full blood work analysis) and then a nutritional response to the condition to prevent recurrences.

The facial paralysis of Bell's Palsy is usually short lived and a recovery back to normal occurs in the majority of patients. Approximately 50% of Bell's Palsy patients will have essentially complete recoveries in a short period of time. Another 35% will have good recoveries in less than a year. About 15% of people will have permanent effects from the condition.

Naturally there are a variety of nutritional and naturopathic, or alternative means, to help hasten recovery from Bell's Palsy...even if you have suffered for a number of years. That's what this book is about. I believe it's the best collection of scientific findings, reporting of current medical protocols, anecdotal evidence, personal experiences of sufferers, literature reviews and plain common sense you're likely to find.

Please read our disclaimer, however, for this educational information is meant to inform, but not intended to diagnose or treat the condition. If you want to try anything discussed within this book, please first check with your physician.

In general, the figures on recovery mean that without any treatment, about 85% of Bell's Palsy patients are expected to recover facial function to either normal or near normal abilities.

It is the remaining 15% of people who need stronger treatment options! Also, you want to do everything in your power to stack the odds in your favor that you'll be in the 85%, and will recover quicker rather than later.

The disorder usually progresses for 7 to 10 days, starting with the sudden onset of facial weakness. Recovery begins at 3 weeks for most (85%) patients, with a full recovery usually by 6 months. Between 4 and 6% of sufferers experience severe deformity of facial muscles with very little return to normal facial movement, and about 10 to 15% of patients will be bothered by an asymmetrical movement of the facial muscles. Recurrence of Bells Palsy, when it happens, may be on the same or opposite side of the face.

All said and done—YES, take hope that you can in all likelihood recover from Bell's Palsy. The famous actor George Clooney, for instance, suffered from Bell's Palsy when he was thirteen years old, and just look at him now!

Bell's Palsy usually is temporary...but for some people that means waiting longer than others. Nevertheless, console yourself in knowing it is usually temporary...especially if you do everything possible to get healthy and shorten its stay.

There is HOPE.

It does take time, however, so that means the challenge of learning patience and doing everything possible to get your body in better shape to help correct any conditions that might have contributed to it in the first place.

There are things you can do NOW to encourage a speedy and FULL recovery, whether or not you've had Bell's Palsy for years or it's a condition of recent onset.

Let's begin.

Chapter 2
The Cause and Progression of the Condition

As stated, the cause of Bell's Palsy, which has been demonstrated in several studies, is thought to be the herpes simplex virus type I which attacks the facial nerve and causes swelling. In a 1995 study, Dr. Shingo Murakami and others determined that the herpes simplex virus (HSV-1) was probably the most frequent cause of Bell's Palsy, possibly accounting for at least 60—70% of cases. Additional research since then has been slowly reinforcing the conclusion. No one knows for certain, but this is the best conclusion so far.

The idea is that the herpes virus, which is latent in the cranial nerves, somehow becomes reactivated and starts replicating within the nerve cells. The virus travels up and down the cells, producing an inflammatory response. The result is inflammation of the nerve and compression, segmental demyelination of the nerve and then nerve paralysis. That paralysis is the outward sign of Bell's Palsy.

The facial nerve that's involved with Bell's Palsy—the 7th cranial nerve, first studied by Sir Charles Bell—is within the fallopian canal in the head, which is close to the internal auditory canal. This area, which has a diameter of approximately .68 mm, is where doctors believe the nerve is being compressed, thus causing the paralysis. Because the compression is caused by inflammation, doctors usually try to treat the condition with anti-inflammatory steroid medications (such as prednisolone or methylprednisolone) and to combat the virus they use anti-viral drugs. Doctors usually feel the optimal "window of opportunity" is about seven days as the best time for starting these medications.

As stated, most people usually awaken from their sleep to find they have Bell's Palsy facial paralysis. Alternatively, another common pattern is that a patient initially experiences the feelings of dry eyes or tingling around their lips, which then slowly or quickly progresses to classic Bell's Palsy paralysis during that same day. Sometimes the symptoms progress much slower and take several days to become recognized as Bell's Palsy.

The degree of paralysis one can expect with Bell's Palsy should peak within several days after the onset on the condition, usually within 48 hours after the sudden onset, and rarely get worse after the two week mark. If your condition deviates from this general pattern by continuing to get worse over time, please see a doctor who may come up with an alternative diagnosis.

Regardless of how it's triggered, you have to think of the onset of Bell's Palsy as an event caused by "trauma to the nerve" and as with any type trauma or injury, you have to remember that healing is to follow, and expect it to follow.

The question is, what can you do to encourage that healing through alternative, naturopathic means?

What can you personally due to ensure that the odds are stacked in your favor for the best, highest or maximum healing outcome possible?

And...if you have suffered Bell's Palsy for a long time—past the normal statistics—what extra steps might you take to encourage that healing to take place if it already hasn't?

Whether your recovery is fast or slow, and whether it's full or partial always depends on the severity of the initial injury and the steps you personally take to do something about it and encourage healing. If the nerve has suffered nothing more than a mild trauma, the recovery from Bell's Palsy can be swift and involve only several days time...or it can take several weeks.

Condition wise, the sequence of recovery is not consistent among patients. For some people their mouth may move before their ability to blink returns; in other cases it will be the eyelids which regain mobility first and the mouth last.

You might start to twitch before you regain facial muscle movements but it doesn't always happen that way. You might experience pain in the areas of the face that are starting to wake up, and then again, maybe not. The sense of taste[2] may start to change as muscle mobility and taste sensations return, or you might not sense any changes in your taste sensations at all.

Time wise, the recovery can be gradual, rapid, and it can hit occasional plateaus. The "average" recovery usually takes between a few weeks and a few months, though many believe this can be speeded up with natural protocols. For instance, many people find that vitamin B12 often cuts recovery time from two-and-a-half months to just two weeks!

Science says that the cranial nerve regenerates (shall we say "heals") at a rate of approximately 1-2 millimeters per day, and studies suggest it can continue to regenerate for eighteen months. Some suggest the figure is even longer....and the alternative protocols we'll spotlight have been found to help people who've had the condition for as long as thirty-five years.

So there is hope...

Basically, what I'm saying is that regardless of your condition, you can usually expect a healing from Bell's Palsy and can work to effect improvements of your appearance beyond the initial time frame of the condition. You just have to decide you're going to do something about it, and do enough of the right things.

Statistics have shown that about 50% of all Bell's Palsy sufferers have complete and spontaneous recovery, without any treatments or interventions, within the first thirty days after the onset of the condition. Another 20% recover between the first and third months. Lastly, between months four and six we usually see another 5-10% of recoveries. So that's a total of 80% of sufferers exhibiting "spontaneous" recovery within six months, and 85% in less than a year.

Of course half a year (six months) or a full year is too long to wait if you can shorten it.

The Bell's Palsy patients who have not completely recovered by the end of six months are often considered "residual," as they are healing too slow. These are the stubborn cases, and these patients advised to go for some form of facial muscle rehabilitation, which we'll get into.

For now, let's proceed to the acute medical treatment usually provided by modern medicine.

Chapter 3
Standard Medical Treatment: Steroids and Anti-Viral Medications

The traditional medical approach to treating Bell's Palsy is to use high dose steroids, such as Deltasone®, methylprednisolone (Medrol®), and prednisolone (Prelone®, Pediapred®). The purpose behind these medications is to reduce the swelling and inflammation of the 7th facial nerve so that the facial muscles can regain their strength.

If your doctor decides to use medication to help relieve the compression, they should be started as quickly as possible. The "window of opportunity" for starting these medications is thought to be the first seven days from the first onset of Bell's Palsy, though of course some doctors continue to prescribe anti-inflammatories for a longer period of time when it appears the inflammation has not subsided.

The first priority in treating Bell's Palsy (or any type of facial paralysis) is to eliminate the source of nerve damage as quickly as possible. A minor compression of a nerve for a short period of time can result in mild, temporary damage. However, as time goes on with constant or increasing compression, damage to the nerve can also increase. That's the reasoning behind the necessity for a quick response with anti-inflammatory drugs.

Doctors will also often prescribe an anti-viral medication such as Acyclovir or Famvir since it is believed that the nerve inflammation is caused by a viral infection, specifically the herpes simplex one virus (Acta Otorhinolaryngal 1988, 446: 114-118). So in effect, when a doctor prescribes Acyclovir, he's treating the condition as if it were indeed caused by herpes simplex.

A typical prescription by a doctor might include Prednisone at 60 mg per day (20 mg t.i.d.) for one week followed by a rapid drop off in dosage, and Famvir in a dose of 500 mg b.i.d. Once again, doctors are the only one who can give these prescriptions. If you have Bell's Palsy, please take any self-help aids under the guidance of a physician as well.

Studies show that the use of steroids is safe in treating Bell's Palsy. As to their effectiveness in improving facial functional outcomes, that's another issue. Some studies conclude there are no appreciable benefits to using steroids at all. Other studies show there are benefits.

Because of the logic behind the approach, most doctors believe that prednisone treatment will help speed recovery and reduce the frequency of a bad result. Prednisone must be given within the first week of facial weakness, in order to be most effective, and I've read in places that some doctors feel it's best to start before day 2 of the condition.

The prednisone dosage is usually 1 mg/ kg of body weight daily for 15 days, tapering to 0 during the next 5 days. Another common practice is just prescribing a dose of about 60 mg per day in a single morning dose, continued for about a week, and then tapering off to nothing at about 10 days. Prednisone mimics cortisol and suppresses immune function, so it can't be administered to patients with existing immune problems.

Doctors also typically use antiviral treatment for herpes simplex in hopes to improve the prognosis of patients (Adour, 1996). The typical protocol is the antiviral medication acyclovir at 400 mg taken 5 times a day for 10 days. Another common option is famciclovir (500 mg tid) or valacyclovir (Valtrex). Once again, your doctor will know the right prescription.

Analgesics such as acetaminophen, aspirin, or ibuprofen may relieve the pain of Bell's Palsy, but patients should talk to their doctors before taking any over-the-counter medicines because of possible drug interactions. Prednisone itself can interact with the following medications to produce side-effects: birth control pills, blood thinners, NSAIDS, ibuprofen, barbiturates, diuretics, acetazolamide, digoxin, phenytoin, rifampin, rifabutin and amphotericin B.

In most cases, deciding to undergo decompression surgery to cure Bell's palsy—in order to relieve pressure on the facial nerve—is not recommended. Serious complications, such as hearing loss, have often been reported. We won't talk about this option because this is book on natural Bell's Palsy helpers rather than surgery, and this surgery is highly controversial.

The Problems With These Medications

As stated, the first problem with using steroids for Bell's Palsy (or any other condition) is they can cause a wide variety of side effects. The known side effects include stomach upsets, mood swings, thrush, irregular periods, weight gain, acne, sweating, fluid retention and depression. However, this is pharmaceutical medicine's first line of defense for the condition. Perhaps the worst thing is the fact that these drugs may not be effective in treating Bell's Palsy at all.

In fact, a recent major scientific review (called the "Cochrane Review") of all the information available on Bell's Palsy treatments concluded, at least, that the steroid treatment does not seem to offer any significant benefits:

"Four trials with a total of 179 patients were included. One trial compared cortisone acetate with placebo; one compared prednisone plus vitamins, with vitamins alone; one compared high-dose prednisone administered intravenously against saline solution, and one, not-placebo controlled, tested the efficacy of methylprednisolone. Allocation concealment was appropriate in two trials, and the data reported allowed an intention-to-treat analysis. The data included in the meta-analyses were collected from three trials with a total of 117 patients. Overall 13/59 (22%) of the patients allocated to steroid therapy had incomplete recovery of facial motor function six months after randomisation, compared with 15/58 (26%)

in the control group. This reduction was not significant (relative risk 0.86, 95% confidence interval 0.47 to 1.59). The reduction in the proportion of patients with cosmetically disabling sequelae six months after randomisation was also not significant (relative risk 0.86, 95% confidence interval 0.38 to 1.98). The trial not included in the meta-analysis showed a non-significant difference in outcomes between the arms....The available evidence from randomised controlled trials does not show significant benefit from treating Bell's palsy with corticosteroids. More randomised controlled trials with a greater number of patients are needed to determine reliably whether there is real benefit (or harm) from the use of corticosteroid therapy in patients with Bell's palsy."[3]

In addition to the Cochrane Review, two papers have looked at the usage of corticosteroids in children with Bell's Palsy and also came to the conclusion of little or no proved benefit:

- http://www.bestbets.org/cgi-bin/bets.pl?record=00778
- Salman MS et al, Should children with Bell's palsy be treated with coricosteroids: a systematic review, Journal of Child Neurology, 2001, 16 (8), 565.

As to the antiviral acyclovir, we know that it may cause jaundice, skin rashes, dizziness, tiredness and kidney failure. A separate Cochrane Review examined acyclovir or valaciclovir for Bell's palsy (idiopathic facial paralysis):

"Three studies met our inclusion criteria, including 246 patients. One study evaluated aciclovir with corticosteroid versus corticosteroid alone, another study evaluated aciclovir alone versus corticosteroid and a further study evaluated valaciclovir with corticosteroid versus corticosteroid alone or versus placebo alone....An analysis was performed on data reported at the end of the study period in each trial. The results from one study four months after the start of treatment significantly favoured the treatment group, whilst the results of the study three months after the start of treatment significantly favoured the control group. The results from the second study at four months showed no statistically significant difference between the three groups....More data are needed from a large multicentre randomised controlled and blinded study with at least 12 months' follow up before a definitive recommendation can be made regarding the effect of aciclovir or valaciclovir on Bell's palsy.

Although a Cochrane Review of the two most common traditional approaches to Bell's Palsy came up with non-conclusive results, interestingly enough a Cochrane Review on an alternative / complimentary therapy for Bell's Palsy—namely acupuncture—states that acupuncture showed some benefit! Acupuncture is the traditional way, within the workings of Chinese Medicine, to treat the condition.

Later we'll discuss acupuncture's use to help with Bell's Palsy, but not for now.

So with that behind us, we will soon step into the realm of what you can do in terms of alternative treatments to help your condition.

But first, we must address a major concern for Bell's Palsy sufferers, which is what to do short term and long term about the inability to blink and readily close your eyes.

Eye protection is priority concern with Bell's Palsy, and I want this book as helpful as possible, I have put this information in a separate chapter by itself.

Chapter 4
Take Care of Your Eyes: AM and PM Remedies

It's not uncommon for Bell's Palsy to affect the eyelids, and since they are the guardians of the eyes, the eyes must still be protected even though the face becomes paralyzed.

The big problem is blinking because facial paralysis of any type can limit a person's ability to blink with ease. When the eyelid is unable to blink or close, tears are not moved across the surface of the eye and it dries out.

And you have to worry about this not just during daytime, but when you're sleeping, too!

Normally we blink every 5-7 seconds. Since your body uses blinking to move tears across the eyes to maintain its moisture, remove external contaminants (pollen, dust, debris, etc.), keep its surface smooth, and deliver nutrients to eye cells as well as remove cellular wastes, a major concern is how to immediately protect your eyes from debris and from drying out when you no longer have this function.

If your cornea dries out and becomes scratched because you cannot blink well anymore, your vision may suffer permanent damage.

I'm going to say this many times: All Bell's Palsy sufferers therefore need to take immediate steps to protect their eyes, and I'll introduce some of the steps that patients have found most effective for this, all of which you should discuss with your doctor. The key, however, is to do something right away.

Usually what happens with most cases of Bell's Palsy is that people are temporarily unable to blink or close their eyelid completely on the affected side of their face. In that case, most people simply need to keep their eyes moistened with special eye drops. They must also use special protection during the day or night to prevent their cornea from drying out or becoming damaged during the recovery period.

Just remember that when the eye dries out because your tearing is no longer being washed across its surface, or when debris gets into the eye and is not washed out by tears, or when you cannot blink away your own tearing, this can lead to eye damage that you should avoid that at all costs. This is the big danger of Bell's Palsy.

With Bell's Palsy, you must continually take care of your eyes until the condition resolves, and quite a few things are possible that will make this quite simple to do. There are both <u>AM and PM solutions</u>: the steps might seem inconvenient at first, but really are quite simple.

Now Bell's Palsy eye problems can involve all sorts of factors. Sometimes the tear glands in the eyes may not be producing enough moisture. For some people the eyes may appear to be tearing excessively, especially while you are chewing. Sometimes it only seems like the eye is producing excessive tears because the tears are just collecting there in the lazy lower eyelid, or continually running out of the eye,[4] rather than being spread evenly over the eye by normal blinking.

Regardless of the cause, take immediate action if your eye feels uncomfortable. A stinging or burning sensation in the eyes can mean your eye has become too dry, even if tears are apparent. So don't let the tears fool you.

The 7th nerve affected by Bell's Palsy does not control vision focus, so if you are experiencing blurred vision, don't ignore it because it may be warning of a dry cornea that needs to be protected.

Daytime Eye Protection

For Bell's Palsy sufferers, the daytime treatment of the eye is relatively simple. In many cases all that is needed to help maintain eye moisture during the day is **artificial tears**, and you can ask any pharmacist for advice on the proper over-the-counter artificial tear drops to try.

Follow the instructions on the label (or given by your doctor), but in general, you apply the artificial tears to your eyes about every 2 hours to keep the eyes moist. Keep them readily available throughout the day...I suggest you buy several bottles so that you can take them with you and have them available wherever you go.

Whenever the drops are not available and whenever you feel the need, you can always use a finger to manually close your eye to moisten it. Don't feel any shame in this if you must do this in public…it's no different than having to adjust a contact lens if something goes wrong. You should always adjust your eyes if they feel dry or uncomfortable. All you have to do is manually blink your eye, using the back of your finger, at regular intervals.

Here's a big word of caution to remember once again: if your eyes feel a stinging or burning sensation then they are probably too dry, even if there are tears in the eyes. And if you are experiencing blurry vision, it may be a warning sign of a dry cornea as well. Let the sensations, and not the presence of tears, guide you as to the identification that a problem exists.

Get proper eye care at all costs!

Now when selecting artificial tears for purchase, I suggest you look for a brand labeled "non-allergic", "preservative free", "for sensitive eyes", and so forth. The preservative thimerosal, which contains mercury (50% by weight), can be a particularly irritating ingredient in eye drop solutions, so that' something to consider. It all depends on your personal sensitivity.

The drugs most commonly used inside the popular over-the-counter eye drops include carboxymethylcellulose (Refresh Plus®, Celluvisc®), polyvinyl alcohol (Murine®, Liquifilm

Tears®, Hypotears®), and hydroxypropyl methylcellulose (LubriTears®, Tears Naturale Free®, Moisture Drops®). Of these brand names to choose from, the most popular brands for sufferers seem to be:

- Bion tears
- GenTeal
- Tears Naturale
- Celluvisc

While these over the counter artificial tear solutions usually help, if stinging or burning occurs with any of the gels or drops, it may mean that you are sensitive to one of the ingredients within them. If that's the case, just try another brand, but try a new brand that is from one of the other main ingredient groups cited, which is the reason they're grouped that way. If that doesn't help, see your ophthalmologist for even more solutions.

In any case, never ignore the symptoms of a dry eye with Bell's palsy. I cannot emphasize this enough.

Now during the day, since the eyes may not close with facial paralysis, you need to protect them from the sun. Sunglasses are a perfect solution which will also help protect your eyes from injury and reduce possible dryness from exposure to the wind. PanOptx Dry Eye / Windless EyeWear has designed fashionable sunglasses for the public that function like a moisture chamber.

You can also wear special protective glasses or an eye patch to protect against dust and debris like pollen and lint. An eye patch will give your eye a rest here and there and that will really help with the fatigue. Your personal ophthalmologist is the one who should be able to provide you with the patch.

Another common option is a "moisture chamber" that will provide you with the same, or even better protection than a patch, and since it's clear it will also allow you to have better vision.

One type of moisture chamber that works quite well looks like a pair of goggles designed for just one eye. There are also moisture chambers that clip onto eyeglasses. Have your optometrist look into this option if it sounds interesting. Several brand names to consider:

- Vision, Inc.'s "Rectangular Moist Eye Moisture Panel" (Eagle Vision Inc)
- Franel Optical Supply's "Moisture Chamber Occluder"
- NitEye Dry Eye Comforter.

An alternative to a moisture chamber is to make your own patch with plastic wrap over your eye, and taped to your face. If you want to do this, try using surgical tape rather than any other type because it will be easier to remove and is gentler on your skin. Vaseline can sometimes be used to hold it in place.

Other than wraparound sunglasses, even swimming goggles are a useful alternative to a moisture chamber. It may sound funny to be using swimming goggles, but they are a really good solution for nighttime eye protection, and also important for the shower.[5] Several popular brands (you can do a web search to find more):

- • TYR Racetech goggles
- • Nike K-6 goggles
- • Speedo Hydroflash goggles

Just remember that all these precautions are to help prevent the surface of your eyeball from drying out. Even if your eye is watering non stop, the best advice is that you still need to use the artificial tears. Of course, whatever route you choose should be discussed with your doctor.

Night Time Eye Protection

For nighttime protection when your eyes will not close, using heavier eye lubricants than the artificial tears (or lubricants combined with an eye patch) is a good solution. However, since sometimes people who choose to use a patch do so incorrectly and end up scratching the eye's cornea while they sleep, a few words of warning are in order. Hopefully your doctor will teach you how to do this, but just in case, here's what you should know.

When you tape the eyelid shut at night to reduce dryness and the risk of injury to the eye, if it isn't done correctly then the eyelid can easily pop open during the night and you can end up rubbing the eye against the tape and scratching it. The result, in this case, can be damage far worse than from not using the tape. Therefore make sure to use a gentle, non-abrasive and easily removed tape (such as paper surgical tape), and learn the correct way to apply it. Your doctor will show you how.

If you do choose to use a patch for your eye, you can add a plastic wrap patch beneath it for added protection should the patch shift position. You might also use an eyeshade over the patch to also help keep it in place. Franel Optical Supply also makes a product called the "Peel-n-Press Occluder" that helps eliminate the chances of the patch moving during the night.

Wearing a pirate's patch may seem romantic when you don't need it, but when you do need it, such as here, it really is an inconvenience. However, the benefit of a pirate's patch is that you can put it on or take it off as you need it, and of course it's supplying the protection you want. In addition, it gives you a way of dealing with public embarrassment.

Yet another popular night time solution is sleeping with swimming goggles while using the gel at night. The goggles form a tight seal that, combined with the gel, keeps the cornea moist. Swim goggles are very hard to slip off, easy to get used to and avoid many of the worries we're discussing.

Here's several popular possibilities for night time gels. Once again, your doctor or pharmacist can advise you on the best options for your situation. The most popular gels include:

- Lacrilube
- ViscoTears
- HypoTears
- Refresh PM—this one has a thinner consistency than the others, making it easier to handle

You can also use these heavier gels and lubricants during the day, rather than just eye drops, when you want more lubrication than eye-drops normally provide. However, because they are thick (gels are thicker than artificial tears is due to the addition of mineral oil), your vision can be a bit blurry when you use them.

Contact lenses

Whether or not you should wear contact lenses when you have Bell's Palsy is something you have to find out from your optometrist or ophthalmologist. They're the ones to best help you decide—don't decide this one on your own.

For instance, on the one hand contact lenses hold water because they are hydrophilic and designed to do so, so naturally you'd think they'd help you. Because they hold water, they can provide a source of moisture directly over your cornea and help protect the eye from debris. There's even something called a "bandage contact lens" that an optometrist can place over your (affected) eye. It's a giant, clear contact lens—without any corrective optical power— that covers the entire eye for protective purposes.

For regular contact lenses, your eyelids are what work to help to keep them held in place. If your eyelids become limp because of Bell's Palsy, contact lenses cannot be worn until you start to regain some of this function. Whether or not a bandage contact lens will work will be up to your optometrist or ophthalmologist to determine.

Another factor to consider is the fact that wearing contact lenses does not replace the need for tears and keeping your eyes moist. Even if things seem perfectly fine, you still need to keep applying plenty of contact lens saline solution or eye drops when you have Bell's Palsy.

At the earliest stages of Bell's Palsy, the eyes can be so dry that it is impossible to keep a contact lens moist for more than a few minutes. If this is the case, contacts cannot be worn, which is another reason to remind you that if you want to wear contact lenses, it's best to consult with your eye doctor for his expert advice and opinion.

The need to protect your vision from permanent damage is so important that it's not wise to make major eye care determinations on your own even if you believe you can manage your own eye care. There is no substitute for professional evaluation and advice. And when your eye stings or burns or feels scratchy or dry, remember it's sending a message.

Other Eye and Facial Options

For the small number of people who have long-term paralysis from Bell's Palsy, there are a variety of treatment options that do no not fall within the alternative treatments field, and go well beyond the intended scope of this book. These are options and procedures you must discuss with your physician. Nevertheless, let me do you a favor by introducing a few of these options in brief.

Botox Injections

For some people, a small dosage of Botox (botulinum toxin) can be injected into their upper eyelid to cause it to droop temporarily, and thus protect the eyes.

Some people use botox to enhance their appearance when suffering from Bell's Palsy residuals because the procedure can change your appearance dramatically. Botox can also be used during facial retraining in order to prevent certain muscles from moving while other muscles are taught to regain their original functions.

Using Botox correctly for Bell's Palsy is a complicated topic and not something to consider immediately, so we'll leave the pros and cons to your attending physician should you not be healing as quickly as you should be.

Punctal Plug Insertion

Punctal plugs can be an effective step for treating moderate to severe cases of dry eye that are unresponsive to artificial tears or ointments. That's why they are sometimes used with Bell's Palsy.

With punctal plug insertion, which is a simple procedure, the tear ducts are partially blocked so that both natural or artificial tears will remain on the eye longer. Punctal Plugs are known to cause very little discomfort (only 10% of people complain about any discomfort), and can be removed with a saline pressure wash. About 40% are naturally lost within six months of insertion.

Another related short term option for plugging the tear ducts (so that tears remain on the eye longer) are self-dissolving collagen plugs, which are effective for about ten days.

Regular punctual plugs are usually made of silicone, but a recent invention by the Medennium Corp ("SmartPlug") a special acrylic polymer material that changes from a rigid solid to a soft, cohesive gel as it warms from room temperature to body temperature. Once again, it can be removed with irrigation.

Facial Retraining

Probably the foremost option you should consider—when the facial muscles are still not responding and the eyelids are still not closing properly after a long period of time—is a form of physical therapy known as "facial retraining."

Also known as "neuromuscular retraining," this physical therapy can help minimize the non-symmetrical appearance of the face that occurs when one side becomes weakened or paralyzed because of a condition like Bell's Palsy. The best explanation of facial retraining therapy is probably found at the website www.bellspalsy.ws/retrain.htm and you are advised to go there for more detailed information.

Don't discount this therapy, as it has a well proven track record in helping the facial nerve recover from non-use or damage. Although a variety of modalities such as acupuncture, chiropractic, myofascial release, electrotherapy, physiotherapy, cranial sacral massage, cranial osteopathy, NCR, IMT and other forms of bodywork massage can be somewhat tempting to the long term Bell's Palsy sufferer, and even though they can help somewhat with improving the appearance of the face and help in regaining muscle mobility, this is the one proven approach I recommend to overcoming the results of facial nerve damage when everything else has failed. People often resist the one thing that will help, and facial retraining does help!

If the facial muscles have been paralyzed for a long time and new nerve fibers grow back during the paralysis connecting to the wrong facial muscle, causing synkinesis,[6] this is the therapy to go for.

Special exercises for Bell's Palsy patients have been developed along these lines to reverse the situation, but you need to find a qualified facial retraining therapist in your area to begin therapy. This will be worth the effort for "residuals" because facial retraining has a long, proven track record in helping to improve muscle mobility even when the therapy is started years after the onset of Bell's Palsy.[7]

Therefore if you are reading this book now after years of Bell's Palsy, and haven't yet tried this, this is something to consider.

The rule of facial retraining is to proceed slowly rather than to push for results too quickly. It takes time to heal and to retrain the muscles. With longstanding cases of Bell's Palsy, you have to slowly recreate the brain-to-nerve-to-muscle connection because synkinesis, cross-wiring, hypertonic muscles and spasms are likely to have developed over time. Muscles need to relearn their old movements, and additionally inappropriate movements that have developed need to be unlearned. Unfortunately, the only way to properly relearn correct muscle reactions is through slow relearning of coordinated actions.

Facial retraining will help correct the synkinesis that sometimes happens to long term Bell's Palsy sufferers. It will also help correct any facial tightness and impaired facial nerve and muscle functions. Most of all, it'll make you feel like you're doing something other than just waiting for the condition to get better.

For the long term sufferer who still has facial paralysis and/or disfigurement, check into this right away. Some of the exercises you would normally practice for facial retraining, under the guidance of a therapist, include:

- Sniffling and wrinkling the nose
- Frowning and drawing the eyebrows downward
- Hardening the chin
- Smile without showing the teeth, and then smile showing the teeth
- Pressing the lips together, puckering and then whistling
- Gently winking with one eye, and then alternating to the other
- Opening your eyes WITHOUT moving the eyebrows
- Raising the eyebrows, holding for a few seconds, and then wrinkling the forehead

For more information, see: www.bellspalsy.ws/exercise.htm

Tarsorrhaphy

A surgical procedure called tarsorrhaphy, which narrows the space between the eyelids by having them stitched together, may also help improve the problem of eye closure in Bell's Palsy. The procedure is also sometimes considered for patients with myasthenia gravis, Grave's disease, Sjogren's syndrome and for stroke sufferers.

In tarsorrhaphy, a surgeon sews just a tiny portion (only a few millimeters) of the upper and lower eyelids together at their outer corners; your eyelashes remain undisturbed. It's a minor procedure done under local anesthesia. The surgery has few risks and complications.

When the stitching is that small (usually under 5 mm), the change in physical appearance is not too noticeable. The change is also comfortable because it's not so large, and you can still maintain good peripheral vision.

Unfortunately, for some people the procedure will not be effective unless a much larger area is stitched, and in those cases the results become noticeable and can interfere in cutting off part of the peripheral vision.

Yet another surgical option—that of elevating the lower eyelid and surgical tightening the lower lid—can help prevent moisture from accumulating between the eye and the lazy (droopy) bottom eyelid. You can read more about this option here: http://www.eyelid.com/paralysis-bell's.html

Gold and Platinum Eyelid Weights

When Bell's Palsy sufferers still cannot close their eyes after a long period of time, another surgical option is to have gold or platinum weights fitted (sewn) into the upper eyelid to help keep the eyelid closed by using gravity.

When sewn into the eyelid, these weights are visually un-detectable...and the lids will still open normally. The smaller weights used for this purpose are not uncomfortable for most people and the gold or platinum materials do not cause irritation to the surrounding tissues because they are highly biocompat-ible.

These weights, if used, are removed as soon as enough nor-mal function returns to the eyelid though in cases of permanent facial paralysis, because they're made of gold they can be left in place indefinitely. Using gold eyelid weights, however, is a surgi-cal procedure, and should be done only after careful consider-ation. The good news, if you choose this route, is that the surgi-cal implant procedure usually takes less than one hour and can be done on an outpatient basis under local anesthesia.

As with any surgery, there can be complications to this procedure such as infections and swelling, but excessive swelling and inflammation or pain after the procedure is usually very rare. Your doctor can explain all the potential ramifications of this type of surgical implantation.

One thing to remember, besides these risks, is the fact that you will still need eye protection while sleeping because the weights work on the principle of gravity; since we sleep in a horizontal position the weights will not help keep our eyes closed while sleeping.

External Eyelid Weights (From the MedDev Corp)

A new development is the availability of removable skin tone, external eyelid weights from a company called Med Dev, available only by prescription. These weights are not inserted into the skin but simply taped on the upper eyelids to make them heavier, which helps with the effort of blinking. To use them, the weights are simply attached with double-sided adhesive tape to the upper eyelid(s) that need(s) them.

MedDev's "Blinkeze External Lid Weights" are made of tantalum, which is a dense metal with high biocompatibility so that the weights don't seem to bother the skin. The way it works is that the weight uses gravity to help gently close the upper eyelid when the wearer looks down, or when the eyelid muscle is relaxed. MedDev offers their External Lid Weights in a variety of skin tones to match people's complexion.

The problem with these weights is that the sticky adhesive can often cause irritation. Although a bit cumbersome, for temporary Bell's Palsy paralysis this is another short-term solution. If someone is going to have weights permanently implanted, this helps them adjust to living with an eye weight prior to implantation surgery and also helps judge the amount of weight necessary for the best effect.

Chapter 5

Methyl Form Vitamin B12 and Other Helpful Nutritional Interventions

Okay, now on to the alternative remedies for Bell's Palsy—stuff that works!

Probably the very first thing a doctor should consider if you are diagnosed with Bell's Palsy is to give you an injection of vitamin B12. That's right—an injection of vitamin B12. This certainly will not hurt, and may indeed help.

In all probability, your doctor will not have heard of this non-pharmaceutical cure. Physicians often don't know about these alternative medicine practices, and aren't taught nutritional practices or interventions in medical school. Their curriculum is all pharmaceuticals, pharmaceuticals, pharmaceuticals.

Nonetheless, this cheap and safe option has lots of research (and reported anecdotal case studies) suggesting that it is the best, first and foremost protocol for a condition where conventional medicine knows no effective treatment.

Let's go into some of this B12 research, which you should take to your doctor.

First, in a 1959 report, patients with Bell's Palsy experienced a complete or almost complete recovery—even if they had had the condition for up to 4 years—within 20 days of receiving daily injections of vitamin B12. In this report, patients were successfully treated for chronic Bell's palsy with vitamin B12 injections of 500 to 1,000 mcg given every one to two days. The recovery of facial nerve function was also reported for long term sufferers when low doses were used!

In more recent trial involving 60 Bell's Palsy patients, the effects of 500 mcg of injected vitamin B12 (in the form of methylcobalamin) given three times weekly for at least eight weeks—were compared with the results from steroid medication, or both. Researchers found significantly faster recovery in the groups given B12 injections with or without steroids, compared to those given steroids alone.

These findings agree with earlier reports on the effectiveness of methylcobalamin injections for Bell's palsy.

What this is actually saying is that vitamin B12 was found to be more effective that steroid treatments in hastening the recovery of the symptoms! And as we'll see, there's ample theoretical evidence as to why B12 can and should work.

So from the 1959 study, patients receiving vitamin B12 recovered after two weeks on average, whereas those on steroids recovered after about 10 weeks. In light of the fact that vitamin B12 is well known for actively protecting nerves, reducing nerve inflammation[8] and reducing the amounts of nerve irritants (such as the toxic chemical glutamate), the results make perfect sense. Take them to your doctor! This is not proof of the effectiveness of B12, even though methyl B12 is used to treat other neuro-pathologies. Nevertheless, since high dosages of B12 don't appear to have adverse side effects, many people opt for "it cannot hurt to try it."

The sources for this information are:

Mitra M, Nandi AK, Cyanocobalamin in chronic Bell's palsy, *J Indian Med Assoc*, 33: 129-131, 1959.
Jalaludin MA, Methylcobalamin treatment of Bell's palsy, *Methods Find Experim Clin Pharmacol*, 17: 559-544, 1995

This is probably one of the first things you should do if you wake up one day with symptoms of Bell's Palsy. Methyl vitamin B12 is incredibly cheap, safe and people often give it to themselves. There's oral B12 available and injectable B12 available, for which you need to consult a physician.

Now a blood test can usually tell you whether your B12 levels are low, but in many cases the test that is used to measure the amount of vitamin B12 in the body is not sensitive enough to detect a deficiency of the vitamin. Nutritionists and naturopaths have known this for years, but it's only recently Florian Thomas, M.D., Ph.D., Laurence J. Kinsella, M.D., associate professor of neurology, and Jamie T. Haas, M.D., a neurology resident, at Saint Louis University School of Medicine[9] have publicly published results showing that the standard test for B12 deficiency—measuring its blood level—may be too insensitive.

So even if the blood work results show your levels are fine, you would be well warranted to ask your doctor for injections anyway due to the successful medical research. I'd do the blood work anyway because it might be able to tell you if something else is going on, and even confirm the choice of the response you take.

As an aside, a variety of other nutritional blood chemistry indicators, first developed by Harry Eidenier PhD (his reference is *Balancing Body Chemistry: Making Sense of Blood Chemistry Results*), can also suggest the need for supplemental B12 when your B12 blood work levels seem normal. For instance:

- When uric acid levels are on the low side in a blood exam (<3.5 for men, < 3.0 for women), this suggests the need for vitamin B12 (and molybdenum supplementation).
- When MCV is elevated (> 89.9) this suggests the need for B12 and folic acid supplementation
- When RDW (red cell size distribution) is greater than 13, this may also suggest B12 anemia.

A deficiency of vitamin B12 is not uncommon, and most people who develop deficiencies do so as a result of malabsorption, meaning that their bodies no longer efficiently extract it from food. It's not only common with those who have little stomach acid, but with vegetarians, macrobiotic dieters and vegans who aren't eating enough vitamin rich foods.

Typically, a deficiency of vitamin B12 usually takes years to develop, which may explain why older people are more susceptible to Bell's Palsy. Because pregnant mothers are using up all their vitamin supplies to nourish their fetus, that may explain their threefold increase in risk, too.

Vitamin B12 deficiencies are normally treated with injections, though recently scientists have found that in some cases oral supplementation can also sometimes correct the deficiency when the oral doses contain more than 200 times the recommended daily allowance (RDA). Some people try to take the healing process into their hands, and do just that.

In fact, Dr. Lisette C. P. G. M. de Groot of Wageningen University in the Netherlands found that daily oral doses of 647 to 1032 micrograms of vitamin B12 appeared to correct normal deficiencies,[10] but these levels are much lower than the ones therapeutically found to help with Bell's Palsy in the studies quoted.

As a background, vitamin B12 deficiency is well proven to contribute to nerve degeneration, which is a tie-in to the assumed causality of Bell's Palsy syndrome. Also, both the injectable AND the oral forms of vitamin B12 have been commonly used to treat many types of nerve disorders.

It is unlikely that oral vitamin B12 would be as effective as the injectable B12 dosages (500 mcg three times a week). However, it's possible to get vitamin B12 in 5 mg lozenges that can be taken up to eight times a day to try to duplicate the result of injectable B12, which is what some people choose to do.

A word about oral forms of vitamin B12...

What you're looking for with oral B12 is not "cyanocobalamin," which is the more common type of B12 you'll find in vitamin supplements. Because you are specifically seeking B12 for a health condition, many alternative physicians advise you to be using methylcobalamin B12 (also known as "methyl B12") because it is more readily absorbed by the liver.

Methyl B12 is a very important neuro supplement that has been safely used for Bell's Palsy and degenerative neurological disorders such as ALS, Parkinson's, multiple sclerosis, etc. It is also known to feed the aging brain and can greatly improve early Alzheimer's symptoms as well as other forms of dementia (even doctors agree on this). All these conditions have to do with nerve degeneration, which is a direct tie-in with Bell's Palsy. Aside from Bell's Palsy specifically, however, vitamin B12 supplementation has been proven to improve cognitive function and help reverse mental impairment in the elderly, who tend to get Bell's Palsy in the first place.

With cyanocobalamin B12, the liver needs to convert it first to the methyl form before it can properly absorb it and much of the needed aspects of the B12 are lost during this process. The liver converts only about 1% of cyanocobalamin into its active methyl form. Evidence indicates that the methyl B12 form of vitamin B12, in addition to having a theoretical advantage over cyanocobalamin and not requiring intrinsic factor, actually has some therapeutic and metabolic uses that the other forms of vitamin B12 lack. Two other forms of B12—adenosylcobalamin and hydroxocobalamin—do not share its many benefits.

The dosage for methyl B12 for nerve recovery is a minimum of 25,000 mcgms[11] under the tongue though practitioners with a lot of experience with Bell's Palsy patients say it really should be a sub-lingual dosage of 40,000 mcgms[12] daily for best results. Methyl B12 is water soluble and difficult to absorb so if you take less than this amount orally, it may not work. Stomach acid usually destroys B12, which is why methyl B12 is taken sublingually under the tongue. In this way it is absorbed directly into the bloodstream, bypassing digestion. Blood tests of B12 indicate that sublingual forms become available about 15 minutes after ingestion, and levels tend to stay elevated for a day.

Some alternative physicians suggest that 40-60 mgs per day should be the standard protocol for nerve regeneration. While the dosages sound high, for vitamin B12 there is no known toxicity. Once again, as with everything in this report, proceed with the advice and under the care of your physician. After things get better, people often reduce the dosage substantially, which is to about 5 mgs per day or less. A blood test or ION panel can help your doctor determine what dosage to be on for long term supplementation.

What is an ION panel and why might it be useful? I know you've probably never heard of one, so here are the facts:

The number of medical conditions managed by, and even reversed by nutritional substances is astronomical. Books and books have been written based on this simple fact.

There are so many conditions that have an underlying cause based on body biochemistry and that biochemistry can be altered, modulated, even "fixed" through the proper form of nutritional supplementation. But how do you guide yourself on what nutritional factors you might be missing and what supplements to take to help fill in the gaps and thus modulate a medical condition?

There is some tendency for Bell's Palsy to run in families, and while scientists look for a genetic basis or predisposition, the condition might actually be due to underlying nutritional factor deficiencies in the diet COMBINED with genetic predispositions to burn up or use those factors more quickly than for others. This makes a lot of sense.

For instance, possessing the genetic predisposition to use up B12 quickly might contribute to the manifestation of Bell's Palsy. A family diet too high in the amino acid arginine might encourage the replication of the herpes virus to levels that cause the condition, and so on it goes. There are so many possibilities no one can list them all.

Sometimes a medical condition simply needs more of a particular vitamin or mineral to become stabilized (or be prevented) because the conditions "burns" it up, and supplying more of that substance helps return things to normal. "Genetic predispositions" are sometimes managed just through this mechanism; it's not the genes themselves, but what you WASH over the genes that causes them to express or not. So feed your body the missing factor and you have a way to affect your health.

Now, Bell's Palsy may indeed be one of these conditions that benefits in this manner, but no one has done the nutritional and blood work studies to find out. Therefore there's nothing I can say on this account EXCEPT…I can teach you how to see for yourself and intervene specifically for any of your own nutritional stores that are deficient and any biochemistry that has gone awry which can be modulated. It might help (then GREAT!) and it might not (in which case you won't be any worse off, but probably helping internal conditions of some sort anyway). Without clear data, nutritional intervention is sometimes like flying in the dark, just as is the practice of traditional medicine at times. This test will give you the data you need to make wise health decisions regarding nutritional supplements.

If through an RBC[13] blood analysis you find that your body is lacking sufficient stores of some particular level of vitamin or mineral, perhaps THAT is contributing to Bell's Palsy or its recurrence…and perhaps then supplementing with that missing factor may help reverse the condition or prevent it in the future. This is especially important to know when you do suffer from a recurrence of Bell's Palsy. What's going on may mean "what's missing inside" that is leading to this predisposition.

It's conjecture at this point, but with nothing available from medical science at this point, this type of information would be useful to you, wouldn't it? In fact, it is the basis of the alternative medicine approach.

When people have high cholesterol, as an example, they take steps to reduce the chances of future cardiac events by supplementing with high doses of folic acid, vitamin B-6 and vitamin B-12 to modulate homocysteine, the "glue" that binds cholesterol plaque to the walls of arteries. If you reduce levels of homocysteine, then less plaque tends to form on arterial walls.

This same type of biochemical detective work is what YOU can do hand-in-hand with a nutritional doctor (or on your own if you're smart enough) once you have information on the various enzyme, mineral, amino acid, and fatty acid levels in your blood, and know how they play a role in various biochemical pathways. Once you see what's deficient and understand how they might play a role in Bell's Palsy, then it's easy to map out a more logical supplementation plan.

Therefore what we're looking for is some deviation in your levels of minerals and vitamins and other factors in your body that might tie in to Bell's Palsy, so here's how you do it: You get a blood test...but not just any old blood test.

You ask your doctor to help you get a _specific_ blood test.

You need to get your doctor to order an "ION panel," which is the least expensive, most comprehensive, and most technically accurate laboratory test I know of to assay your vitamins, minerals, fatty acids, amino acids, organic acids, heavy metals and more.

If you've got a disease then something is off internally, and this panel will help tell you about your underlying biochemistry.

Then you can go about the most scientific nutritional modulation of your condition.

A full ION (individual optimal nutrition) panel includes:

- Functional Deficiencies Markers for Vitamins B1, B2, B3, B5, B6, B12 and Folic Acid
- Vitamins A, E, B-Carotene and Coenzyme Q10- (serum)
- Essential Elements- (plasma)
- Amino Acids—(fasting plasma)
- Fatty Acids—(plasma)
- Organic Acids—(overnight urine)
- Lipid Peroxides (TBARS)- (serum)
- Homocysteine- (serum)

With this type of information and the logical tie-in to what we know about Bell's Palsy or suspect, it's a lot easier to come up with a natural protocol that might help with the condition.

Always the idea of nutritional therapy is to fix the underlying deficiencies, to build bridges where there is none, to maximize the chances for healing to take place. With knowledge such as the following, you'll see that nutritional intervention is rarely a one-supplement sort of thing.

Don't Take B12 Alone—Combine Supplementation With Other B-Vitamins

If you elect to take vitamin B12, that's not the only B-vitamin you should take. Traditionally, any nutritionist or naturopathic doctor worth their salt will tell you that the B-vitamins work as a group, and if the level of one is low you should probably be supplementing them all.

In particular, Vitamins B1, B2 and B6 (in addition to folic acid and vitamin B12) tend to work together and are particularly effective at boosting other factors that nourish the nerves. They are commonly taken together when there is any form of nerve damage or brain failure in an individual.

You really need a qualified nutritionist or nutritional physician to recommend the appropriate short term emergency dosages of the B-vitamins for Bell's Palsy. However, the super dosages for these vitamins in a case of Bell's Palsy have been suggested as:

- Vitamin B1 (Thiamine) is 50 mg three times a day
- Vitamin B2 (Riboflavin) is 50 mg three times a day
- Vitamin B6 (Pyridoxine) is 50 mg—100 mg three times a day

In one study of another B-vitamin—namely vitamin B-3 (naicin)—74 consecutive Bell's Palsy patients were treated with niacin at a dose of 100-250 mg with "excellent results" noted in all patients within 2 to 4 weeks.[14]

So how much of these vitamins is enough?

The methyl B12 or injectable B12 levels have already been explained, but as to the other B-vitamins, it simpler just to find a high dose B-vitamin tablet from a reputable company (Thorne, NOW, Jarrow, Supernutrition, etc.) and take that rather than individual amounts of the various B-vitamins. In my opinion, the best brand or manufacturer for B vitamins is probably Freeda Vitamins. I've had supplement manufacturers tell me that they won't even add B-vitamins to their line because they are so fragile, but in tests comparing various producers, Freeda B-vitamins ranked well above any other competitors because of their unique production process. So for any B-vitamins, I always recommend the Freeda brand just as I always recommend Jarrow for CoQ10.

B-vitamins are water soluble, so you tend to excrete the extra B-vitamins that you don't need through your urine. Over a very short period of time, there shouldn't be any problem of toxicity though you have to watch the levels of B6 and niacin you might take for longer periods of time.

Nonetheless, the niacin study is just further evidence that you should be taking a high dosage B-vitamin, and a multivitamin/multi-mineral complex in general with adequate amounts of zinc, if you have Bell's Palsy. In many cases, conditions like Bell's Palsy occur in the first place because there was some underlying sub-clinical vitamin or mineral deficiency that lead to some chain reaction of events making the onset possible. If that's so, a daily vitamin-mineral supplement may help to prevent recurrence.

In many medical conditions, after pharmaceutical treatment or even surgery you may still have all sorts of underlying nutritional deficiencies that are contributing to the condition in one way or another (the "weakest link" theory) and the only way to correct those deficienices is with supplementation. That's the basis of the alternative medicine approach—find those underlying causes or weakness and fix them.

If you don't know what to specifically supplement, which can be determined through the ION panel results,[15] a very good multi-vitamin/multi-mineral supplement is the best shot gun approach available. Personally, after years in the nutritional field trying many different multibrands with clients, I favor any of the multi-vitamin supplements made by SuperNutrition of California. But if you are just going to take a single B-vitamin or B-complex for some specific health condition you know you have, Freeda is the brand I like best. For a specific methyl B12, you must search on the internet for an available brand.

The studies cited say that vitamin B12 injections if possible, although costly, are a proven way to quickly speed an end to the condition if you act fast enough. Past that initial period of shots many people supplement with sublingual methyl B12 and adjunctive extra B-vitamins along with a multi-vitamin and multi-mineral going forward. This is common sense, not medical advice or treatment. Most naturopaths and nutritionally oriented physicians suggest that you should be taking a multi-vitamin/multi-mineral anyway so this is simply restating the obvious.

The methyl B12 may perhaps deliver the greatest response you can get using a single supplement, and I know of cases where it has turned off the pain of Bell's Palsy overnight. Since it's also used with peripheral neuropathy, which causes numbness, it might help with other underlying neurological conditions.

This is the key supplement if you're lazy and only want to take one. Depending upon how much money you want to spend and how many pills you want to take, I'd next go with the high dosage B-vitamins together with the multivitamin. You can also supplement with acetyl-l-carnitine and other nutrients, but this is the first tier of priority items.

An ION panel can tell you what other vitamins and minerals you might be missing that might have contributed to the disease, and only with such information in hand can you make a more informed decision about what you should do.

Acetyl L-carnitine

Another nutrient, acetyl-L-Carnitine (ALC) has also been found to improve the symptoms of Bell's Palsy.[16] While not as many studies have been done on using acetyl-l-carnitine for Bell's Palsy, the finding makes sense because ALC is an anti-inflammatory compound used in a variety of neurological diseases including nerve injury and nerve weakness, which is what occurs in Bell's Palsy.

ALC is known to stabilize the membrane of nerves, reduces damage done by free radicals, helps preserve nerve cell function and is involved in the production of nerve growth factors in the brain.[17] These functions, together with its anti-inflammatory effects (which is why doctors prescribe the steroids), make it a reasonable and logical supplement possibility, together with the B-vitamins, when you suffer from Bell's Palsy.

There's another reason behind the possible helpfulness of using ALC as well. One of the components of ALC is the amino acid lysine, which is well known for preventing the outbreak of the herpes simplex virus. In a variety of studies, lysine has been shown to reduce the recurrence rate and symptoms severity of herpes outbreaks, so herpes sufferers are often advised to supplement with lysine capsules. One possibility of supplementing with ALC is that it will be broken down into lysine, which will attack HSV (herpes simplex virus) just as would Acyclovir…and will contribute to directly reducing inflammation itself.

This actually leads to some dietary tips behind preventing future reoccurrences of Bell's Palsy…and maybe from the following facts you might be able to trace a dietary incident that might have been a precursor of the onset.

A few years ago, researchers discovered that the herpes virus—which is thought to be responsible for Bell's Palsy—needs the amino acid arginine in order to grow. The foods high in arginine concentration include chocolate, peanuts, almonds, seeds, cereal grains, gelatin, and raisins…so you would be well advised to stay away from these 7 foods if you have Bell's Palsy. Once again, you might also choose to supplement with lysine during this period as well.

The amino acid lysine competes with arginine for absorption and entry into tissue cells. And when lysine is present, it inhibits the growth of HSV by knocking out arginine. This makes a diet high in lysine and low in arginine a useful tool in managing HSV infections.

In a recent study, participants consumed large amounts of lysine (about 1 gram three times each day) while restricting food sources of arginine. A significant number of participants (74%) noticed an improvement in their HSV infections and a decrease in the number of outbreaks. Lysine supplements (as opposed to foods high in this nutrient) can also play an important role in staving off and reducing the severity of herpes-related cold sores. Lysine supplements may even prevent HSV outbreaks in chronic sufferers.

As a result of this information, we can summarize as follows:

- Acetyl-L-carnitine supplements may help Bell's Palsy patients
- Bell's Palsy sufferers should probably stay away from foods high in arginine, namely chocolate, peanuts, almonds, seeds, cereal grains, gelatin, and raisins
- At the onset of Bell's Palsy, supplementation with lysine may help to combat the herpes virus and thus combat Bell's Palsy

Histamine and MSM

Another study has shown that MSM (Methyl-Sulphonyl-Methane), which is an anti-inflammatory nutritional supplement containing sulfur, can also help the pain of Bell's Palsy at a dosage of 500 mg three times a day. But this is not a first tier supplement to try unless you have nerve pain or if an ION panel or hair analysis shows sulfur as an underlying deficiency.

Our nerves are comprised of connective tissue which is dependent on sulfur based amino acids. MSM, containing sulfur, has been shown to inhibit pain impulses along nerve fibers, decrease inflammation, dilate blood vessels to increase blood flow, soften scar tissue, aid hair, skin, and nail growth, produce an immune normalizing effect as in auto- immune disorders. Basically, it reduces muscle spasm and pain, and so much so that US Olympic training athletes commonly use 8,000-10,000 mg daily to avoid muscle soreness, for muscle strains, tendonitis, and athletic injuries. That's the story behind MSM.

Low-dose histamine therapy, which has been prescribed by otolaryngologists primarily to treat Bell's Palsy,[18] has also been used to successfully treat the inflammation of Bell's Palsy in the past (Ear, Nose and Throat Journal 1999, 78/5 (366-370). Since histamine is not generally available and your doctor is not likely to prescribe it, we won't spend much time on it other than to say I've seen it help many cases of Multiple Sclerosis for prolonged periods of time.

Consider this a topic needing further research rather than something to jump onto when you're first diagnosed with Bell's Palsy. However, there is one further point: carnosine is a nutrient which helps regulate histamine production, so some people take carnosine supplements when they get Bell's Palsy because histamine isn't available in tablet form.

ATP

In yet another study (Eur. Arch. Otorin. 1991, 248(3):147-149), the chemical adenosine triphosphate (ATP) was used together with the B-vitamin group to see whether this combination had a significant impact on the recovery from Bell's Palsy. In past studies, for herpes doctors have injected the body with AMP (adenosin-5'-monophosphate, an intermeditae in cellular metabolism and nucleic acid sysnthesis) because they noticed elevated levels of ATP and reduced levels of AMP in blood samples, and found it helped clear up herpes lesions and prevent recurrences.

ATP, however, was supposedly chosen in the Bell's Palsy because it is an essential agent involved in producing energy in the cells, but along those lines the study should probably have looked at CoQ10 in conjunction with these supplements as well since it, too, is involved in cellular energy production.

Anyway, the results of the study showed that 100% of those patients who had a partial paralysis of the nerve, and up to 87% of those who had full paralysis, recovered completely. In contrast, only 67% of patients treated with steroids recovered.

You can boost your production of ATP by taking a supplement such as "Mitochondrial Resuscitate," which contains the B-vitamins riboflavin, thiamin and acetyl-l-carnitine hydrochloride. Even though studies have not yet been done, I would also take CoQ10 (coenzyme Q10) along with it if I were to choose this course of action, which is not a top priority. Zinc, by the way, is also used to combat herpes and speed nerve growth, and it is recommended as well.

For The Pain of Bell's Palsy
Rather than MSM, a topical cream that you might first want to try on your face for the pain of Bell's Palsy, and which has been proven safe and effective in clinical studies for periph-

eral neuropathy nerve pain, is "Neurogen PN." It's manufactured by Origen Biomedicinals and made from Geranium oil and associated botanical oils.[19]

It's also been reported that Far Infrared Treatments can also help relieve the paralysis, discomfort, pain and ill effects of many patients who suffer with Bell's Palsy. With FIR treatments, you just aim an FIR lamp at the affected area of bare skin, from about 16 inches away, for 30-60 minutes, 1-3 times daily. Basically it's a type of moxibustion, which is a Chinese acupuncture procedure of burning herbs over trigger points in the body. However, in this case the heating is done with light.

Some doctors will recommend, as a self-help program of physical therapy, that a patient apply gentle heat to the facial muscles to help reduce any pain, such as using microwavable pads. This is a similar alternative. Doctors commonly suggest moist heat packs, like Thermophore, for sciatica pain but I have not yet heard of it being used for Bell's Palsy.

Typically, people most often turn to acetaminophen, aspirin, or ibuprofen to relieve the pain of Bell's Palsy but you must check with your doctor on their usage. Many individuals have reported that upon taking methyl B12 there was spontaneous disappearance of their pain, so once again the priority of possible supplementation stays the same.

Chapter 6
Acupuncture

I previously wrote that a Cochrane Review on a number of studies that used acupuncture for Bell's Palsy,[20] which is the traditional Chinese Medicine means for dealing with the condition, actually found that acupuncture showed treatment benefits... whereas steroid usage did not. This, of course, will naturally depend upon the skill of your acupuncturist. Acupuncturists are like doctors, lawyers and accountants. Assuming your condition is treatable, you go to a good one and get a good result, go to a bad one and get a bad result. It's important to check out the reputation of your acupuncturist before undergoing treatments.

A variety of other studies have also claimed that acupuncture therapy speeds recovery from Bell's Palsy and/or facial paralysis as well:

Zhang Y. Clinical experience in acupuncture treatment of facial paralysis. J Tradit Chin Med 1997;17:217–9.

He S, Zhang H, Liu R. Review on acupuncture treatment of peripheral facial paralysis during the past decade. J Tradit Chin Med 1995;15(1):63–7 [review].

Yuan H, Zhang J, Feng X, Lian Y. Observation on electromyogram changes in 93 cases of peripheral facial paralysis treated by point-through-point acupuncture. J Tradit Chin Med 1997;17:275–7.

Zang J. 80 cases of peripheral facial paralysis treated by acupuncture with vibrating shallow insertion. J Tradit Chin Med 1999;19:44–7.

He L, Zhou D, Wu B, Li N, Zhou MK. Acupuncture for Bell's palsy. *The Cochrane Database of Systematic Reviews* 2004, Issue 1. Art. No.: CD002914.pub2. DOI: 10.1002/14651858.CD002914.pub2.

J Tradit Chin Med 1999 Mar;19(1):44-7. Zang J, Second People's Hospital, Kaifeng, Henan Province.

Acupuncture may or may not help your condition.[21] It actually depends on how long it's been since the onset of Bell's Palsy, along with the skill of your acupuncture practitioner. If it's been less than 4 weeks since the onset of Bell's Palsy, acupuncture often shows results within 2 weeks time whereas if acupuncture treatment is started after 4 weeks, the results take longer to show and may not be as good.

Having lived in Asia for many years, I can attest to the fact that you can experience remarkably different results with different clinical therapists practicing the same technique simply because of a difference in skill levels. Some may use electro-stimulation, or micro-stimulation, and others will only use traditional needles.

Acupuncture falls into this category of therapies where the results highly depend upon the skill of the practitioner and how quickly you decide to try the treatment.

Basically, Bell's Palsy is one of those conditions where patients usually DO BENEFIT from acupuncture, and starting acupuncture treatments sooner is better than later.

The only way to know if acupuncture will work for you is not to debate about it, not to think it's something strange, but just try. First find an acupuncturist who's had prior experience with Bell's Palsy, try 2-3 sessions (one isn't enough), and see if it helps. That's how you'll know.

Western medicine believes that acupuncture works because of some sort of nerve enervation that it doesn't yet understand, whereas Chinese medicine states that it works by regulating the chi (qi) or life force of your body, directing it to areas where it may have become deficient (i.e. paralysis).

Regardless as to how it works, if it works then it works… and it's simply up to you to see if it works for you. Most people who've tried acupuncture with Bell's Palsy have experienced some degree of help with their treatment.

I've heard of people getting good results with acupuncture for up to two years after the onset of the Bell's Palsy, so it's still an option for long time sufferers even though the best results come from starting it sooner.

For long time sufferers of facial paralysis, the really important therapy I urge you to try is not so much acupuncture but facial retraining. You can spend all the money you want on a variety of therapies, and they'll all help somewhat, but this one will really help the long term sufferer of "residuals."

Chapter 7
Homeopathy

There's also the possibility that homeopathic remedies—which also work at the level of the chi or life force of the body—can help someone with Bell's Palsy. While it's best to find a skilled homeopathic doctor to help you with something as serious as Bell's Palsy, the www.abchomeopathy.com site actually has an online self diagnosing computer program[22] that will teach you how homeopaths determine which homeopathic remedy has the best chance of helping you.

The standard rules of homeopathy are to select a remedy to try that most closely matches your symptoms. What's unusual in homeopathy, which also works on the life force aspect of your body, is that "your symptoms" therefore also can include emotional tendencies and all sorts of indications that might not seem related to the condition, such as whether you like spicy food, sleep on the left side of your body, become emotionally irritated quite easily, like ice cream and so on.

Typically for self-treatment, a lower potency (6X or 6C, 12X or 12C, 30X or 30C) homeopathic remedy should be tried; instructions are usually printed on the label that you should follow.

The standard principle used by most homeopathic physicians is that you take one dose of a suggested remedy and then wait for a response. If an improvement is seen in your condition, then you continue to wait and let the remedy work. If, on the other hand, the improvement lags significantly or has clearly stopped, another dose of the remedy may be ingested.

Most remedies come in bottles with instructions that will tell you to avoid taking the remedies at the same time as coffee, tea or other stimulants, and that you should let the remedy dissolve in your mouth under your tongue rather than swallow it. You also should not touch the homeopathic pills because that contaminates them.

The frequency of dosage for a homeopathic remedy varies according to the individual and the condition, which is why only an experienced homeopathic doctor can BEST determine the best remedies to try. Sometimes a dose should be taken several times an hour; other times a dose may be indicated several times a day; and in some situations, one dose per day (or less) can be sufficient.

If no response is seen within a reasonable amount of time, a homeopath will tell you that you need to select a different remedy.

As with picking any sort of physician, to pick a good homeopath you must take into consideration their years of experience as well as any prior experiences they've had for treating Bell's Palsy.

Your homeopath will ask you a series of question from which they'll be able to determine the correct remedies to apply, and for information-sake some of the possible, and most often recommended homeopathic remedies for Bell's Palsy that will probably be considered include:

Aconitum napellus—this homeopathic remedy is often used when facial paralysis occurs after exposure to wind or cold air. In general, the emotional tendency of the patients responding best to this remedy are those who are usually a bit fearful and agitated.

Agaricus—a remedy used in Bell's Palsy when grimacing and/or twitching occurs on one side of the face while the other half feels stiff. People needing this remedy tend to be emotionally excitable and suffer deep worries (in general) about their health.

Cadmium sulphuratum—a remedy used under the following conditions of facial paralysis: often one of the eyes cannot be completely closed, the mouth may appear distorted, and the condition sets in after an exposure to wind of some type (in Chinese, a "wind invasion").

Causticum—this is used when the paralysis developed slowly and gradually, usually on the right side rather than the left. The patient finds it difficult to open and closer their mouth and may often accidentally bite the sides of their mouth or tongue.

Cocculus—this remedy is often used for one-sided facial paralysis, wherein pain/tension is felt on the other unaffected cheek, especially when opening the mouth.

Dulcamara—a remedy used when a person has one-sided paralysis of the face and finds it difficult to speak. This remedy is often used for a variety of health conditions that develop after exposure to damp and cold, such as rainy weather, which may mark the onset of the condition. Those who need this remedy often suffer a tendency toward back pain, sinusitis and allergies.

Nux vomica—this is a popular remedy applied for all sorts of health conditions, but in terms of paralysis, it's usually prescribed for people who tend to be irritable and slightly hypersensitive. If they feel cramping or constricting sensations, rather than numbness, this is another indication.

Platinum (Platina)—this remedy is used when someone suffers a painless paralysis of the face. Usually, you pick this remedy if one eyebrow seems raised and the patient experiences numbness in other parts of the body, including lips and cheeks.

I consider homeopathic remedies a very useful thing to try at the first onset of Bell's palsy. The reason is that they are extremely cheap ($5-6 per remedy typically), easy to take, usually won't hurt you in any way, and can be added on to any other of the treatment protocols we've gone over without interfering with that protocol.

They are the type of adjunctive alternative therapy that won't hurt and can only help—IF the right remedy is chosen. That requires a very skilled homeopathy practitioner.

Maybe you'll be lucky enough that your indications are so clear that the right remedy just pops out at you after reviewing our list and the information on remedies that you can find on various websites. Nevertheless, the best person to prescribe a homeopathic remedy, along with the correct dosage, is a skilled homeopath with many years experience, and they can usually be found on the web or through your local health food store or newspaper. Good ones are not cheap, but time is also of the essence and you want to minimize your chances of long term problems. You want everything in your favor to help get over Bell's Palsy quickly.

The short set of possible remedies I've supplied can certainly get you started researching the possibility of homeopathic help to shorten the length of your symptoms. The thing to do is get started as soon as possible and to remember as clearly as possible any weather or other conditions that preceded the onset of the disease.

Just as I asked you to consider whether any high arginine content foods may have preceded the onset of Bell's Palsy, you must also try to remember if any of the unusual "indications" identified by homeopathy apply to your case as well.

If family and friends read the various homeopathic indications, they can often better identify your emotional tendencies (indications) rather than you yourself, and that's always a plus helping the homeopath pick the right remedies.

Chapter 8
Other Treatment Alternatives

Hyperbaric Oxygen Therapy

Hyperbaric oxygen therapy (HBT) is an alternative medical procedure that in a well controlled study,[23] has produced a faster recovery rate (22 days versus 34 days) for Bell's Palsy patients than the use of steroids.

In hyperbaric oxygen therapy, a patient is placed inside a pressurized chamber where they breath 100% pure oxygen at pressures up to three times greater than normal atmospheric pressure.

The problem with this therapy is that it's expensive, not readily available, and not something you'll likely encounter. Nevertheless, I'm reporting on it for the sake of completeness.

Biofeedback

Biofeedback techniques (using simple electronic devices to measure and report information about a person's biological system) have been reported to help limit the deterioration of muscle function and speed recovery in Bell's Palsy:

Biedermann HJ, Inglis J. The restoration of control in facial muscles affected by Bell's palsy. Int J Psychosom 1990;37:73–7.

Lobzin VS, Tsatskina ND. The adaptive biological control system with electromyographic feedback in the treatment of Bell's palsy. Zh Nevropatol Psikhiatr Im S S Korsakova 1989;89(5):54–7 [in Russian].

Ross B, Nedzelski JM, McLean JA. Efficacy of feedback training in long-standing facial nerve paresis. Laryngoscope 1991;101:744–50.

However, a controlled trial of patients with chronic facial paralysis (including some with Bell's palsy) found that using a mirror as the feedback mechanism was just as effective as a mirror plus electrical biofeedback for improving facial symmetry and muscle function.

In other words, if you just use a mirror to watch your motor facial pattern through exercises and reinforce the proper responses, this simple technique is just as good as the results from biofeedback.

Basically, there are a number of facial exercises you can do to help improve Bell's Palsy on your own but the best therapy, in my estimation, is neural reprogramming.

Chiropractic and NeuroCranial Restructuring

Many Bell's Palsy sufferers find that chiropractic treatments can be quite helpful with the condition, but the usefulness of the procedure varies because of the differing skill levels of chiropractic practitioners and differing severity levels of patients. Nevertheless, it's something to look into.

What I consider even better than chiropractic treatments are NCR "neurocranial restructuring treatments"...a form of manipulative therapy developed by Dr. Dean Howell. The procedure is painless—I've had it done several times myself just for the "natural face lift" benefits—and involves inserting a deflated balloon in the nose and inflating it briefly. This lifts the sphenoid bone, upon which all other bones in the head rest, and when they are released the compressed bones and muscles in the face restore themselves to more optimal positions.

This can not only help in improving the symmetry of appearance where chiropractic or acupuncture can do nothing, but might also help decompress the 7th cranial nerve AND restore some degree of muscle function.

Doctors trained in the technique[24] are rare but they do commonly treat people with Bell's Palsy, so it's worthwhile to get into contact with them to see what can be done. Many DCR trained doctors are also naturopaths who can offer adjunctive therapies and protocols to help resolve the condition.

For example, one naturopathic doctor told me that *treating his Bell's Palsy patients homeopathically for pesticide exposure seemed to produce the greatest improvements in the condition.* Since there is a great tie-in between pesticide exposure and Parkinson's disease, where there is actual destruction of the nerves in the brain, an analogous irritation of the seventh cranial nerve due to similar agencies may have merit.

Until a few years ago, doctors would recommend surgical procedures to decompress the facial nerve, which involved very serious risks and is not now recommended. However, this idea of decompressing the nerves might actually be accomplished as a natural by-product of this painless two minute procedure since it readjusts the positions of cranial bones and facial muscles that may impinge upon the cranial nerve. You never know.

Often people turn to plastic surgery when there are long term residuals of Bell's Palsy, but this is a procedure that might actually help with muscle function as well as appearance, where-as cosmetic surgery only improves appearance alone. No studies have been done on this, and the reports vary, but it's something you should look into.

Conclusion: Natural Alternatives Priorities

All in all, the natural treatment therapies for acute Bell's Palsy can be reduced to the following:

- Protect the eyes
- Vitamin B12 shots or methyl B12 oral tablets
- Supplement with extra B-vitamins and a multi-mineral, multi-vitamin formulation; an ION panel can give you guidance as to any deficiencies that need to be corrected that might have contributed to the condition
- Homeopathic remedies
- Acetyl-l-carnitine

- Avoid arginine foods; supplement with lysine
- Acupuncture
- Neurocranial Restructuring

For longer term sufferers:

- Undertake vitamin B12 shots or consume methyl B12 oral tablets
- Supplement with extra B-vitamins and a multi-mineral, multi-vitamin formulation; an ION panel can give you guidance as to any deficiencies that need to be corrected that might have contributed to the condition
- Undergo facial retraining
- Acupuncture
- Neurocranial Restructuring

For the pain of Bell's Palsy, methyl B12 can sometimes end it in one day. Otherwise, Neurogen PN, MSM and the Far Infrared treatment are viable options to check out.

Remember that getting over Bell's Palsy takes time, and time means PATIENCE. Yes there is hope, especially if you select to intervene nutritionally, as explained.

Also, no matter how bad the condition is or how long you've had it, there is always hope as several studies have shown.

Normally doctors don't know anything about natural cures and naturopathic protocols, even when there are medical studies as we've shown, so you're many steps ahead of those who choose to do nothing. Congratulations on being smart enough to educate yourself about your condition, and possibly take the necessary steps at self-help that modern medicine won't teach you about.

The best thing you can do in getting well is acting quickly, and if this book has helped you at all, please send me an email letting me know.

God's speed in getting well, and God Bless.

Chapter 9
Frequently Asked Questions

What is Bell's Palsy?

Bell's Palsy is condition of partial paralysis of the face due to trauma of the 7th cranial nerve. Though not proven with 100% certainty, it's thought to be caused by the herpes simplex virus attacking the nerve, although there are other possible causes as well.

The condition is not permanent, not fatal, not contagious and is not related to stroke. Worldwide statistics set the frequency at approximately .025% of the population. Those who contract Bell's Palsy usually return to normal within a few weeks and can return to normal activities any time they feel ready.

How Sure Can We Be That A Condition Diagnosed as Bell's Palsy Really is Bell's Palsy?

Facial tumors, various cancers and autoimmune conditions can also cause a facial palsy (paralysis) that is sometimes misdiagnosed as Bell's Palsy. Bell's Palsy is often diagnosed through a process of elimination that discounts these other conditions, which is why it's important to be checked out by a qualified doctor. The distinguishing characteristic of Bell's Palsy is that the facial paralysis comes on suddenly.

How is it Normally Treated by Conventional Medicine?

Conventional doctors normally treat Bell's Palsy with antiviral medications and high dose steroids for inflammation. The most important personal treatments focus on protecting the eyes.

The facial paralysis of Bell's Palsy can inhibit your eyelids from blinking freely. Since the body uses blinking to keep the eyeballs moist and to wash away wastes and debris (as well as deliver nutrients), it's important to protect the eyes from drying out. A variety of methods include artificial tears, eye gels, special glasses and eye patches.

Will Acyclovir or Prednisone, Which Are Normally Prescribed by Doctors, Cure Bell's Palsy?

There is no known "cure" for Bell's Palsy although there are a number of natural ways to help speed recovery from the condition, as mentioned in this book. Acyclovir is an antiviral medication used to treat the herpes virus, which is thought to be the cause of Bell's Palsy. Prednisone is a steroid anti-inflammatory medication doctors use to treat the inflammation of the cranial nerve. A number of studies have questioned whether there is any positive benefit to this practice.

Will Alternative or Complementary Medicine Practices Help Bell's Palsy?

Absolutely. There are a number of studies confirming the usefulness of complementary practices, including the use methyl of vitamin B12 and acupuncture, to help shorten the lifespan of the condition and help with recovery. This book contains all sorts of helpful therapies that sufferers have found useful.

Should Bell's Palsy Sufferers Be Concerned About Muscle Atrophy?

Not usually. It takes a longer time for the muscles to begin atrophying than it usually takes for recovery. A variety of facial muscle retraining therapies are also available for stubborn Bell's Palsy conditions. Acupuncture, which is the Chinese treatment of choice for the condition, can also help keep the muscles "alive with energy."

How Long Does It Normally Take to Recover?

Most patients will recover within a few weeks; most within a three month period regardless of whether or not they receive the standard medical treatment. About 85% of Bell's Palsy patients are expected to recover facial function to either normal or near normal abilities. My personal opinion is that naturopathic therapies can definitely stack the odds in your favor for a quick and full recovery.

Can Bell's Palsy Recur?

Yes, the best information estimates the recurrence rate at around 5-9%, with a period of ten years (on average) between recurrences. This suggests performing a full nutritional workup (ION Panel) to see if there are deficiencies of any vitamins or minerals contributing to the inability to combat the herpes virus that typically accounts for the disease, and if any deficiencies may be contributing to the inability to get well soon.

Steps to prevent recurrence might include a low arginine, high lysine diet, and continual supplementation with the necessary B-vitamins and zinc.

What Conditions Increase the Chances of Contracting Bell's Palsy?

Both older and younger individuals can contract Bell's Palsy, though younger patients usually recover quicker. The male/ female rate of Bell's Palsy incidents, as well as its occurrence rate in various races, is also approximately equal. There is also an equal chance of the condition being just mild or severe. Other conditions increasing the risks for Bell's Palsy:

- Diabetics
- Women in their last trimester of pregnancy
- HIV/Aids, sarcoidosis and other immune compromising conditions (Lyme disease, Mononucleosis, Guillain- Barre Syndrome, Heerdfort's Syndrome) increase the odds of facial paralysis occurring and recurring.

Does Bell's Palsy Always Occur on the Same Side of the Face?

The percentage of left or right side cases of paralysis is approximately the same. Even for reoccurrences, the percentages for left-sided or right-sided facial paralysis remain approximately equal. It is possible, though rare, to contract Bell's Palsy on both sides of the face (bilateral Bell's Palsy), but this happens in less than 1% of all cases.

Does Bell's Palsy Affect Any Other Areas of the Body?

Bell's Palsy does not affect any other areas of the body with paralysis. If any other parts of the body become paralyzed, weak or numb, then Bell's Palsy is not the cause of the symptoms.

How Did the Condition Get Its Name?

The condition is named in honor of Sir Charles Bell. Bell was a 19th century Scottish surgeon who first studied the 7th cranial nerve and its enervation of the facial muscles.

Chapter 9
Helpful Links

Best Single Site on Bell's Palsy:
http://www.bellspalsy.ws/

Best Summary of Clinical Treatment:
http://www.neuroland.com/cn/bells.htm

Best Forum—"Brain Talk":
http://brain.hastypastry.net/forums/index.php

Endnotes

1   Named after Scottish surgeon Sir Charles Bell.

2   Whenever anyone loses the sense of taste, you must check for zinc deficiency. Study after study shows that zinc supplementation will often bring a sense of taste back to normal functioning levels, especially in seniors who have lost the sense of taste for years. There is also a variety of very good nutritional reasons to supplement with zinc to fight the herpes virus, and to promote the healing of your nerves.

3   Cochrane Database Syst Rev 2002;(1):CD001942.

4   A condition called "crocodile tears," which often occurs from the onset of Bell's palsy or during recovery.

5   You don't want shampoo running into your eyes, so try switching to gentle, "no tears" baby shampoo during this period if your eyes are not closing properly.

6   If your nerves are damaged or muscles are paralyzed, the brain may wrongly re-wire the nerves in the region as they heal, resulting in unintended movements along with voluntary ones, such as your eye closing when you smile etc. Once again, please see http://www.bellspalsy.ws/retrain6.htm for a deeper explanation of synkinesis and facial re-training.

7   Vitamin B12 therapy does as well, which we'll discuss shortly.

8   Altern. Med. Rev. 1998,3(6):461-463

9   http://www.sciencedaily.com/releases/2004/10/041030213126.
      htm

10   The current RDA for vitamin B12 is 3 micrograms per
      day.

11   25 mgs per day

12   40 mgs per day

13   RBC stands for red blood cell.

14   Arch Otolaryngol 68: pp.28-32, 1958

15   How do you order the ION Panel? Through MetaMetrix
      Labs at 800-221-4640. It's a $1200 value of tests which
      only costs around $600.

16   Neurol. 1997,12(1):23-30

17   Ann. N. Y. Acad. Sci. 2001, 939:162-178

18   It has often been cited as a possible cure for multiple scle-
      rosis, as well, when taken in low doses.

19   The manufacturer is Origin BioMedicinals Inc. in Hali-
      fax, Nova Scotia, Canada B3J 1N7. www.myFootShop.com
      sells it.

20   Allen D et al, Aciclovir or valaciclovir for Bell's Palsy (idio-
      pathic facial paralysis), The Cochrane Database of System-
      atic Reviews 2004, most recent substantive amendment
      January 2004

21   A typical treatment protocol can be found at: http://gan-
      cao.net/ht/bells.shtml

22   http://www.abchomeopathy.com/go.php

23   Racic G, Denoble PJ, Sprem N, et al. Hyperbaric oxy-
      gen as a therapy of Bell's palsy. Undersea Hyperb Med
      1997;24:35–8.

24   http://www.ncrdoctors.com/doctors_list.htm

Made in the USA
Coppell, TX
26 July 2024

35226527R00056